MAYBE it's MALS

Workbook

Median Arcuate Ligament Syndrome

Is your diaphragm getting on your nerves?

By Laurie Krause

Pharmacist, MALS Caregiver & MALS Patient

Co-Founder of MALS Awareness

Edited by Makanda

Copyright 2025 by Laurie Krause

ISBN: 979-8-218-71124-5

Table of Contents

Introduction *5*

How to Use This Book *7*

MALS is a vascular compression syndrome. *9*

Diagnosing MALS *11*

Your Symptoms *12*

The Doctor Might Ask: *13*

Common Comorbidities with MALS *13*

Symptom Diary *15*

Have you had any of these common GI procedures? *21*

What medical issues have been ruled out? *23*

Your Medication List *25*

Common Drugs Prescribed for MALS Symptoms *28*

Food Tracking *31*

Food Diary *32*

Your Care Team *39*

Medical History at a Glance *43*

Insurance Information *53*

After Diagnosis *54*

Surgeon List *55*

Questions for the Surgeon Interview *59*

My MALS *63*

Hospital Go-Bag Packing List *69*

Your Diagnostic Journey *73*

Artistic Side View *75*

Artistic representation of MALS anatomy *77*

About the Author *81*

Introduction

Diagnosing MALS (Median Arcuate Ligament Syndrome) can be a long, drawn-out process. It usually starts with eliminating the more obvious gastrointestinal (GI) issues that could be causing symptoms. MALS might go unrecognized on ultrasounds and computerized tomography (CT) scans because the radiologist was not asked to look for a vascular compression.

The purpose of this workbook is to aid you in the collection of information about your medical journey so that you can refer to it when your doctor asks questions. Quick answers, in an organized manner, will lead to more efficient conversations about MALS. This is not a book offering medical advice, but rather organizational suggestions with a few lists of symptoms, treatments, and drugs related to MALS to help trigger the patient or caregiver's memory for a complete history. This easy-to-read history can avoid time-consuming and costly repeating of tests and drugs. The symptoms point to the GI tract so concrete evidence of normal GI tests are important clues that show this is not a GI problem, but rather a vascular compression problem.

My daughter's journey with MALS took three years to diagnose because MALS was not on anyone's radar. As soon as we learned about MALS and found a vascular surgeon with MALS experience the answers appeared and made sense.

Now that MALS is on your radar, creating a clear medical history could be the next step in finding the right doctors to consider this diagnosis. If you need more copies of the forms you may want to deconstruct this book, make copies, and put it into a three-ring binder. I hope this becomes a tool that serves you on your medical journey.

How to Use This Book

1) Take the time to organize your medical history so that you can find the answers quickly. You might want to add tabs to your favorite pages. Think about the questions a new doctor might ask:
   "When was your last…"
       Endoscopy
       Period
       Thyroid Check
   "What surgeries have you had?"
   "Have you tried _____ drug?"

2) Take this book with you to your appointments, but don't expect the doctor to take the time to glance at more than a few pages. If your doctor is not familiar with MALS, then the next two pages offer a very brief description to jar their memory.

3) Your thorough history may help the doctor connect the dots to MALS, and if you are complex, with more than one syndrome/disease, then a detailed history will help to peel back the layers. For example: I had a friend get diagnosed with MALS, but still had extreme diarrhea. Her food diary held the answers; apples gave her diarrhea because she could not digest them properly.

4) For more in-depth information about MALS I recommend this book:
       Median Arcuate Ligament Syndrome
       A Comprehensive Guide
       By Dr. M.E. Barbati

MALS is a vascular compression syndrome.

The Median Arcuate Ligament of the diaphragm creates an arch in the diaphragm for the aorta to pass through. When a person has the anatomy of MALS, the ligament is too low, compressing the **artery** and **nerves** to the upper GI tract, they may have barely any symptoms until a triggering event inflames the nerves. A finicky stomach can turn into severe pain. Some people have nausea and/or vomiting.

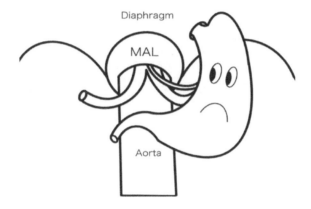

MALS symptoms show up in the digestive tract, often sending patients to GI doctors.

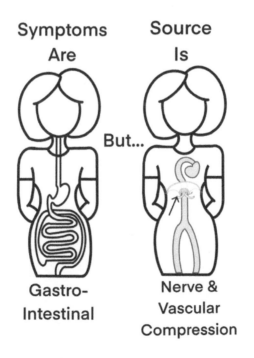

Diagnosing MALS

- **Rule out other GI issues.**

- **Epigastric pain** on examination. (Pushing on the area below the breast bone results in excessive pain. As MALS progresses referred pain spreads, but this is the pain source).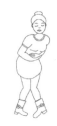

- **Abdominal Duplex Doppler Ultrasound.** (Shows the artery is compressed and the velocity of blood flow through the celiac artery is faster upon exhale.)

- **Imaging** (CT, CTA or MRI, MRA) of the abdominal arteries. "Exhale for MALS" - Images taken during an exhale can make the compression more obvious.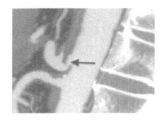

- **Celiac Plexus Block.** If the anatomy of MALS is causing the symptoms, the block will temporarily make the symptoms go away.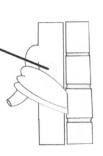

Your Symptoms

Where is your pain?

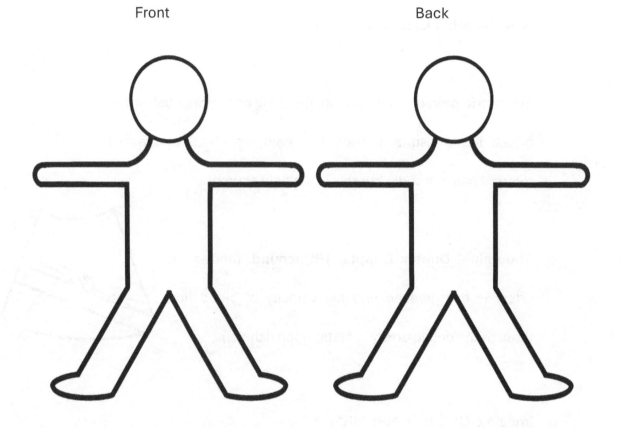

Front   Back

Do you have any of these common symptoms?

- Nausea?
- Vomiting?
- Pain after eating?
- Pain after exertion?
- Early fullness when eating?
- Fatigue after eating?
- Postural change dizziness?
- Blood pressure swings

The Doctor Might Ask:

o   When did the abdominal pain start?

o   Does the pain come and go or is it constant?

o   Is the pain worse after eating or exercise?

o   What relieves the pain?

o   Have you lost weight unintentionally?

Common Comorbidities with MALS
(Have you been diagnosed with any?)

o   Postural Orthostatic Tachycardia Syndrome (POTS)

o   Dysautonomia

o   Ehlers-Danlos Syndrome (EDS)

Symptom Diary

Symptom(s)	Date-time-location	Notes on the last 2 to 8 hours*
Nausea and Pain	05/20/25 5pm at a friend's home.	Started before dinner (strong food smell) Bumpy 2-hour ride in truck at noon. 6am dry toast. 1pm soup.

*Notes may include food ingested, new spices, stress levels, odd smells, changes in deodorant, shampoo, or cleaning supplies. Locational oddities (rocking train, harsh office lights, airplane cabin, etc.)

Symptom Diary

Symptom(s)   Date-time-location   Notes on the last 2 to 8 hours*

*Notes may include food ingested, new spices, stress levels, odd smells, changes in deodorant, shampoo, or cleaning supplies. Locational oddities (rocking train, harsh office lights, airplane cabin, etc.)

Symptom Diary

Symptom(s)Date-time-locationNotes on the last 2 to 8 hours*

*Notes may include food ingested, new spices, stress levels, odd smells, changes in deodorant, shampoo, or cleaning supplies. Locational oddities (rocking train, harsh office lights, airplane cabin, etc.)

Have you had any of these common GI procedures?

Date	Test	Location	Results

- X-Ray of the abdomen
- Endoscopy
- HIDA Scan
- Ultrasound
- CT scan or MRI scan
- Colonoscopy
- Gastric emptying test
- Abdominal Migraine test
- Pill Camera
- Exploratory surgery
- Gall bladder removal
- Appendix removal

What medical issues have been ruled out?

Date   Issue   Notes

-
-
-
-
-
-
-
-
-
-
-
-
-
-
-

Your Medication List

Current Medications (strength and directions):

Drug Allergies – Type of Reaction:

Discontinued Medications - Explain Why.

Common Drugs Prescribed for MALS Symptoms
Drugs do not fix MALS

Anti-Nausea Drugs:
- Zofran (ondansetron), (less popular: granisetron, dolasetron, palonosetron)
- Transderm Scope (scopolamine)
- Compazine (prochlorperazine)
- Phenergan (promethazine)
- Reglan (metoclopramide)
- Vistaril (hydroxyzine)
- Aprepitant (less popular: Fosaprepitant, Rolapitant)

Also Helps with Nausea:
- Haldol (anti-psychotic)
- Thorazine (chlorpromazine, anti-psychotic)
- Zyprexa (olanzapine, anti-psychotic)
- Seroquel (Quetiapine)
- Remeron (mirtazapine (anti-depressant)
- Dexamethasone (steroid)
- Ativan (lorazepam, anti-anxiety)
- Xanax (alprazolam, anti-anxiety)
- Valium (diazepam, anti-anxiety)
- Librium (chlordiazepoxide)
- Bentyl (dicyclomine, anti-spasm)
- Hyoscine (hyosyamine, anti-spasm)
- Cannabis (dronabinol, nabilone)

Non-prescription Nausea Items:
- Emetrol
- Bonie (meclizine)
- Dramamine (dimenhydrinate)
- Benadryl (diphenhydramine)
- Ginger
- Mint
- Iberogast
- Dandelion Root
- Vitamin B6
- Magnesium soaks

Stomach Acid Reducers
- Prilosec (Omeprazole)
- Nexium (esomeprazole)
- Protonix (pantoprazole)
- Aciphex (raberazole)
- Prevacid (lansoprazole)
- Dexilant (dexlansoprazole)

Pain Relief Drugs
- Magic Mouth Wash (lidocaine + Benadryl + Dimetapp)
- Carafate
- Gabapentin
- Pregabalin
- Amitriptyline
- Opiates
- Ketamine
- Cymbalta (duloxetine)
- Tylenol (acetaminophen)
- Motrin (Ibuprofen)
- Aleve (Naproxen)
- Pepto Bismol

Misc. Drugs
- Inderal (propranolol, test for intestinal migraine)
- Depakote (test for intestinal migraine)
- Nitroglycerine (test for esophageal spasms)
- Trazodone (treat esophageal spasms)
- Buspar (treat esophageal spasms)
- L-Glutamine suppliments (Leaky Gut Syndrome)
- Probiotics

30

Food Tracking

Safe foods:

Foods that cause GI distress:

Food Diary

Date:

| Food item | immediate symptoms | one hour later | much later |

| Food item | immediate symptoms | one hour later | much later |

| Food item | immediate symptoms | one hour later | much later |

| Food item | immediate symptoms | one hour later | much later |

| Food item | immediate symptoms | one hour later | much later |

| Food item | immediate symptoms | one hour later | much later |

| Food item | immediate symptoms | one hour later | much later |

| Food item | immediate symptoms | one hour later | much later |

Food Diary

Date:

Food item	immediate symptoms	one hour later	much later
Food item	immediate symptoms	one hour later	much later
Food item	immediate symptoms	one hour later	much later
Food item	immediate symptoms	one hour later	much later
Food item	immediate symptoms	one hour later	much later
Food item	immediate symptoms	one hour later	much later
Food item	immediate symptoms	one hour later	much later
Food item	immediate symptoms	one hour later	much later

Food Diary

Date:

| Food item | immediate symptoms | one hour later | much later |

| Food item | immediate symptoms | one hour later | much later |

| Food item | immediate symptoms | one hour later | much later |

| Food item | immediate symptoms | one hour later | much later |

| Food item | immediate symptoms | one hour later | much later |

| Food item | immediate symptoms | one hour later | much later |

| Food item | immediate symptoms | one hour later | much later |

| Food item | immediate symptoms | one hour later | much later |

Food Diary

Date:

| Food item | immediate symptoms | one hour later | much later |

| Food item | immediate symptoms | one hour later | much later |

| Food item | immediate symptoms | one hour later | much later |

| Food item | immediate symptoms | one hour later | much later |

| Food item | immediate symptoms | one hour later | much later |

| Food item | immediate symptoms | one hour later | much later |

| Food item | immediate symptoms | one hour later | much later |

| Food item | immediate symptoms | one hour later | much later |

Food Diary

Date:

Food item	immediate symptoms	one hour later	much later
Food item	immediate symptoms	one hour later	much later
Food item	immediate symptoms	one hour later	much later
Food item	immediate symptoms	one hour later	much later
Food item	immediate symptoms	one hour later	much later
Food item	immediate symptoms	one hour later	much later
Food item	immediate symptoms	one hour later	much later
Food item	immediate symptoms	one hour later	much later

Food Diary

Date:

Food item	immediate symptoms	one hour later	much later
Food item	immediate symptoms	one hour later	much later
Food item	immediate symptoms	one hour later	much later
Food item	immediate symptoms	one hour later	much later
Food item	immediate symptoms	one hour later	much later
Food item	immediate symptoms	one hour later	much later
Food item	immediate symptoms	one hour later	much later
Food item	immediate symptoms	one hour later	much later

Your Care Team

Doctor_____

Specialty_____

Phone_____

Location_____

Doctor_____

Specialty_____

Phone_____

Location_____

Doctor_____

Specialty_____

Phone_____

Location_____

Doctor_____

Specialty_____

Phone_____

Location_____

Doctor_____

Specialty_____

Phone_____

Location_____

Doctor_____

Specialty_____

Phone_____

Location_____

Doctor_____

Specialty_____

Phone_____

Location_____

Doctor_____

Specialty_____

Phone_____

Location_____

Doctor_____

Specialty_____

Phone_____

Location_____

Doctor_____

Specialty_____

Phone_____

Location_____

Your Care Team

Doctor_____

Specialty_____

Phone_____

Location_____

Doctor_____

Specialty_____

Phone_____

Location_____

Doctor_____

Specialty_____

Phone_____

Location_____

Doctor_____

Specialty_____

Phone_____

Location_____

Doctor_____

Specialty_____

Phone_____

Location_____

Doctor_____

Specialty_____

Phone_____

Location_____

Doctor_____

Specialty_____

Phone_____

Location_____

Doctor_____

Specialty_____

Phone_____

Location_____

Doctor_____

Specialty_____

Phone_____

Location_____

Doctor_____

Specialty_____

Phone_____

Location_____

Medical History at a Glance

An organized timeline can produce fast and effective communication. Each column is a month and the number is the day of the month, followed by the medical event (Test, surgery, ER visit, office appointment, etc.).

Example: Jan 5th vomiting started. Feb 2nd I had an endoscopy.

January	February	March	April	May	June
5) vomiting	2) endoscopy	3) PCP	6) ER	9) neuro	2) PCP
7) PCP	5) PCP	14) GI Dr.	7) PICC	10) CT head	5) Pain Psyc
12) X-Ray	9) G. Empty	16) Colonosc.	8) hospital	20) EEG	12) ER
12) ultrasound	26) Migraine	17) Pain Psyc	9) hospital	25) nero	12) hospital
25) GI Dr.			10) NG tube	15) Migraine	13) hospital
			26) PCP		14) Hospital
					20) GI Dr. #2
					24) CT abdomen
Phenergan Sup			~~Prilosec~~	~~Imitrex tab~~	Reglan
Prilosec	~~Amitriptyline~~		Nexium	Imitrex Inject	Prednisone
Zofran	Imitrex				

Drugs can be listed at the bottom. Women might add first day of menstrual cycle each month.

Tips: You may create in-depth pages for yourself, and a second set of pages with just the highlights to communicate with the doctors. For example, I removed the office visits from the highlight sheet to reduce visual clutter. Also, add any prior surgeries as footnotes in order to have the dates available.

Finally, I usually wrote down my questions for any office visit on a fresh copy of the current six-month calendar, and as the doctor answered our questions or gave us advice I added the information. Later, I consolidated my notes for a six-month period to one page.

Jan 7-Dr. K saw Makanda for vomiting. Tried Magic Mouthwash in office. Gave rxs and referral to GI Doc.

Jan 12-Ultrasound seemed painful- Ask Dr. K if this is normal.

Medical History at a Glance

January	February	March	April	May	June

Medical History at a Glance

July	August	September	October	November	December

January	February	March	April	May	June

July	August	September	October	November	December

Medical History at a Glance

January	February	March	April	May	June

July	August	September	October	November	December

Medical History at a Glance

January	February	March	April	May	June

July	August	September	October	November	December

52

Insurance Information

Fill in the lines below or tape a photo-copy of the card front and back on top.

The insurance carrier is :_____

Card holder name:_____

Patient is: Cardholder or Spouse or Dependent (circle one).

Member ID number:_____

Group number:_____

BIN number:_____

Telephone number:_____

Website:_____

    User name:_____

    Password:_____

I found the insurance website helpful when I wanted to review the medical claims the insurance company had processed. I could clearly see when deductibles were met and what medical bills were on the horizon. Plus, the claim history was very helpful when I first put together my daughter's medical history. Each medical event had an insurance claim, so the claim history gave me an itemized medical history.

A Call Log may be helpful if you are calling your insurance for help:

Date:_____ Name_____Topic_____

Date:_____ Name_____Topic_____

Date:_____ Name_____Topic_____

Date:_____ Name_____Topic_____

After Diagnosis

Once a MALS diagnosis has been made, you may need to educate some members of your care team about MALS. Your path to wellness may still be a struggle if your care team is doubtful about the diagnosis. The simple drawings I've included in the back of the book may be helpful when explaining your understanding of MALS. They make a great starting point for discussions with the surgeon too, as they are easy to add additional markings to explain anatomy and the surgical process.

Choosing a surgeon may be based on MALS experience, surgical approach, geographic location, or insurance coverage. The following pages are for collecting information on the surgeons. Then there are two pages of questions suggested by the members of MALS Awareness. Some people choose just a few of the questions to ask, some people read down the list and some people give the written questions to the doctor. You will know the best approach for your communication style.

Surgeon List

(The working list of surgeons to research)

Name	Phone	City, State	Specialty
Dr. Bill Jones	(555) 555-1111	Seattle, WA	Vascular surgeon, Robotic

<u>Notes:</u> 1/10/25 called office (Susan) taking new MALS patients. Needs Image disc and celiac plexus block results. Offered to refer to pain clinic for block. Booked 3 months out.

1/11/25 called insurance company (Richard) verified this surgeon is in the network and covered by insurance.

1/12/25 Posted on MALS Awareness Group asking for other members who have gone to Dr. Jones.

    Jane Doe responded: good experience.

    Sue Smith: 2 weeks out of surgery. Good hospital experience.

    Fred Jones: 6 years post-surgery. Success!

Surgeon List
(The working list of surgeons to research)

Name   Phone   City, State   Specialty

Notes:

Name   Phone   City, State   Specialty

Notes:

Name   Phone   City, State   Specialty

Notes:

Surgeon List

(The working list of surgeons to research)

Name   Phone   City, State   Specialty

Notes:

Name   Phone   City, State   Specialty

Notes:

Name   Phone   City, State   Specialty

Notes:

Questions for the Surgeon Interview
Developed by Members of MALS Awareness

Do you consider MALS a vascular compression AND nerve compression issue?

How many MALS surgeries have you performed?

What is your success rate?

What is your surgical approach? (Robotic? Laparoscopic? Open?)

Do you clip or trim away the ligament?

Do you touch the nerves? (Cauterize or dissect away from the artery?)

Will you verify my artery is open with normal velocity of blood flow before closing?

What is the plan if my artery recompresses?

Will I have an epidural?

Do you use staples, sutures, or glue on the incision?

Will I have a PCA pain med pump?

Will I have a catheter?

Will I have an NG tube when I wake up?

When will I be allowed to eat?

What is your post-op care plan?

How long is the average hospital stay?

What is your pain management protocol after surgery?

How long will I be on pain meds?

Discharge pain meds will be for ____ days?

How long will I need a caregiver?

Is PT recommended after surgery?

When can I go back to school/work?

How long do you provide follow-up care?

Will you communicate care plans to my PCP?

My MALS

I felt the needle go into my back near my bra line to the right of my spine; there was pain, then pressure, then nothing. I had never felt nothing. The second needle went in on the other side, and I was more receptive to the pain because it led to the feeling of nothing. When they rolled me back to my husband, I had tears rolling down my cheeks.

"Are you alright?" He asked.

"Apparently, I've had a stomach ache for fifty-eight years," I answered in shocked surprise. "I can't remember a time when I've felt nothing."

My GI tests started at seven years old and showed I was normal. I overheard the doctors, teachers, and relatives telling my Mom to force me. Force me to drink milk. Force me to go to school. Force me to be quiet. Speaking about the pain made me a liar. Everyone's response to my truth taught me to be quiet and ignore the pain. Tuck the sensation away so others won't notice.

Now that I am older, sixty-six as I write this, I believe everyone knows someone with a stomach ache. That's why I want to tell our story.

In 2013, my daughter's stomach problems were "triggered". Makanda (rhymes with Amanda) was twenty-three and starting law school. A bulging disc in her lower back and an undiagnosed teratoma tumor on her ovary created tremendous pain in her abdominal area until one morning, the vomiting started. Urgent urping, burping, and dry-heaving exhausted her. As a pharmacist, I felt like a member of her care team and researched her symptoms. The nausea and vomiting had "turned on", and I needed to help her find a way to turn it off.

From our experience, the first encounter with the GI doctor was the most genuine. The doctor believed they would find the source of the distress and their concerns were authentic. But then tests came back negative. The stomach and intestines were healthy. The gallbladder, pancreas, and liver were perfect. This was the turning point from belief to disbelief. Conversations became stilted. Doctors curated their words to deliver the unpleasant messages of doubt; they considered us to be unreliable narrators.

Makanda's first GI doctor ran all the tests, and then he told us it was not a problem with her GI tract and referred us back to her primary care physician. But, all of the symptoms were GI-related, so she was sent to another GI doctor, then another, and another.

She took a leave of absence from school and had her spine fused and the teratoma removed, but the stomach ache continued. The nausea and vomiting consumed her life. They placed feeding tubes up her nose and then directly through her abdominal wall, but each one became too painful to use. Our Seattle doctors were stumped. So we flew across the country to a famous clinic in Minnesota to see yet another GI doctor.

I met Darlene and Vanessa in the hotel's laundry room across from the clinic. I was moving my wet clothes to the dryer when my thoughts became a passionate prayer: please help us find answers.

Then, a woman asked, "Is this washer free?" Her voice seemed familiar, and I looked up expecting to see someone I knew, even though we were thousands of miles from home. That's when I saw Darlene for the first time. She felt familiar and comfortable as if she was my best friend. But I didn't have any friends left after two years of caregiving. I'd pushed everyone away. My friends had opinions and unsolicited advice that made me withdraw into the foxhole I'd dug to keep my daughter safe.

When we compared experiences, we joked that her daughter had POTS (Postural Orthostatic Tachycardia Syndrome) with a side of GI issues, and my daughter had GI issues with a side of POTS. For the next eight days, we got together every chance we could. It was lovely to have someone who just understood without explaining everything. Even after they left, Darlene would text me daily to share our updates.

Makanda was diagnosed with visceral hypersensitivity and told she might never eat by mouth again. We returned to Seattle with a new intestinal feeding tube, which became hypersensitive after a month. That's when her last GI doctor —there were seven total— decided Makanda was afraid to eat and placed an eating disorder diagnosis in her file without telling us. As my daughter starved, the medical staff treated us like incompetent fools. They lied to me about drugs, revised her history, and refused to acknowledge her pain. They were gaslighting us to avoid confrontation.

Then, Vanessa was diagnosed with MALS (Median Arcuate Ligament Syndrome). I had never heard of MALS, a vascular compression disorder where the diaphragm (the Median Arcuate Ligament) sits too low and compresses the nerve bundle to the stomach. As Darlene searched for information, she recognized the symptoms in Makanda. This coincidence just seemed too good to be true. By this time, it had been three years, and I was an exhausted advocate who was numb. I had just warned my relatives that things were bleak for Makanda, and I was starting to fear the worst.

I'd lost all hope for a cure, and communicating with the care team was crazy-making. When I told Darlene I could not afford to chase another diagnosis or to get my hopes up once more, she coaxed me into trying again and said, "I will carry the hope for you."

Darlene found a surgeon with MALS experience and forged the path to Connecticut for Vanessa's diagnosis and surgery. Three weeks after Vanessa's surgery, they were still in Connecticut, staying longer than necessary to be there for Makanda's diagnostic block and surgery. Darlene carried the hope until I could see for myself that this was the answer for Makanda. Immediately after surgery, she could eat once more.

Right there in the hospital room, we envisioned a social media community called MALS Awareness so that other caregivers and patients could connect and share resources: two moms with a passion for finding others with undiagnosed MALS. Currently, it takes an average of three years of suffering to find the correct diagnosis, and we would like to bring MALS into the light so that radiologists, ultrasound techs, and GI doctors look for this compression syndrome routinely.

Two years into Makanda's recovery, it was my turn when my nausea switch was flipped, and I woke up vomiting. The emergency room ordered a CT scan, and the radiologist did not look for MALS. Still, I had learned enough to mail my image disc to Connecticut to be diagnosed with this congenital anatomy. I flew to Connecticut for the diagnostic block (a celiac ganglion block) that gave me relief from a life of stomach pain. Then, my MALS surgery took that daily pain away. If Vanessa had been diagnosed quicker, I shudder to think of what would have happened to Makanda. Darlene will tell you it was all part of a bigger plan—a Miracle. I agree. Vanessa saved Makanda. Makanda saved me. Now, we are working to save thousands more. After all, everyone knows someone with a stomach ache.

-Laurie

LaurieKrause.net

To find a community of people with MALS experience:

MALSawareness.com

Facebook: MALS Awareness Page (public).
          MALS Awareness Community Group (patients and caregivers).

Instagram: @MALSawareness

My Notes on Caregiving

The patient is the narrator. The caregiver is the witness.

The patient must first explain the MALS experience. When bystanders are trying to understand the magnitude of the situation, they may look to the caregiver to validate what the patient is saying. When anyone (doctors, nurses, or family members) challenges your patient's narration, be sure to make it clear that you believe the patient.

Present a united front.

Sort out any disagreements in private. Showing doubt in public will undermine your patient's request for help. Most illnesses are invisible and require trust in the patient's narration. Do not promote distrust.

Do not smooth things over to get along.

If your patient's distress makes others uncomfortable, it is not your job to downplay the situation. When a patient is crying for help, you should not be shushing the patient for the comfort of others.

Shut down any gossip claiming a person is looking for attention.

This behavior is judgmental and dismissive toward your patient. A good advocate will not "go along to get along" on this topic.

No poking.

Please don't poke at your patient to get them to shift their mood. Sick folks don't have the energy for a physical tickle in the side or any good-natured verbal poking. Asking your patient to lighten their mood for your comfort can harm your long-term relationship. Offer situational improvements and let the mood lift naturally.

Hospital Go-Bag Packing List

- This workbook (or medical history, doctor's names, medication list, etc.)
- Insurance card and ID
- Nausea meds (Sea Bands, mints, ginger chews, preggie pops, lemon drops, etc.)
- Birth Control Pills/Critical Meds (you may stay longer than expected)
- Pen and paper for taking notes
- Extension cord
- Phone charger
- Spare battery or battery pack
- Electronics (tablet, laptop, or gaming device) charger, earbuds
- Toiletries
- Hair products (comb, dry shampoo, scrunchies, clips, etc.)
- Glasses or contacts
- Warm comfort top (hoodie, sweater, etc.)
- Pillow for comfort
- Underwear
- Caregiver change of clothes
- Projects (knitting, drawing, reading, etc.)
- Drinks & snacks for caregiver

She's Just Seeking Attention

When I was a child, the grown-ups told my mother I was seeking attention by pretending my stomach hurt. They made my mother choose between believing me or believing the adults. When the doctors could not find the source of my pain, my mom was caught in the middle of everyone's opinions. I learned to be quiet for the comfort of others.

When my child developed MALS pain out of the blue, I respectfully believed her, and I chose her version of the story every time.

Here are a few of my thoughts on the subject of seeking attention:

- I found that chronic illness could be lonely for the patient and the caregiver. I did not seek attention lightly because it often came packaged with judgment.
- My daughter made jokes about feeding tubes to make others more comfortable with the elephant in the room and to lighten the mood, but then she was accused of seeking attention with her jokes.
- Before the MALS diagnosis, when my daughter was told she would not eat regular food again, I drew cartoons of strong, capable people with feeding tubes. Then a pain psychologist accused my daughter of negatively seeking attention by identifying too strongly with the drawings.
- We joined communities of sick people on social media. I wanted to connect myself and my kiddo with others who "just got it." There was always someone who commented that they were just seeking attention. But, I was happy they had put themselves out there for us to find and identify with.
- I wanted doctors to care. Yes! I wanted them to pay close attention.
- I wanted to explain myself to friends so they would understand. Yes! I wanted their compassionate attention.

Now, I want to tell others about MALS. Yes! I am seeking attention.

Your Diagnostic Journey

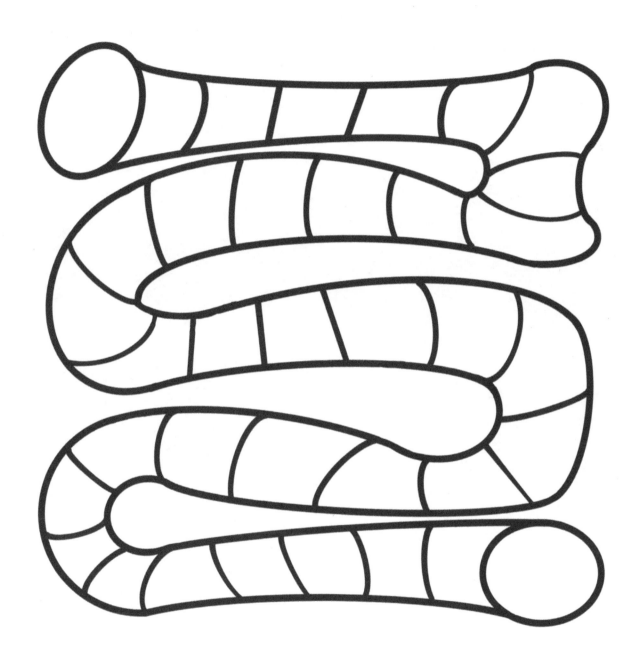

Maybe it's MALS

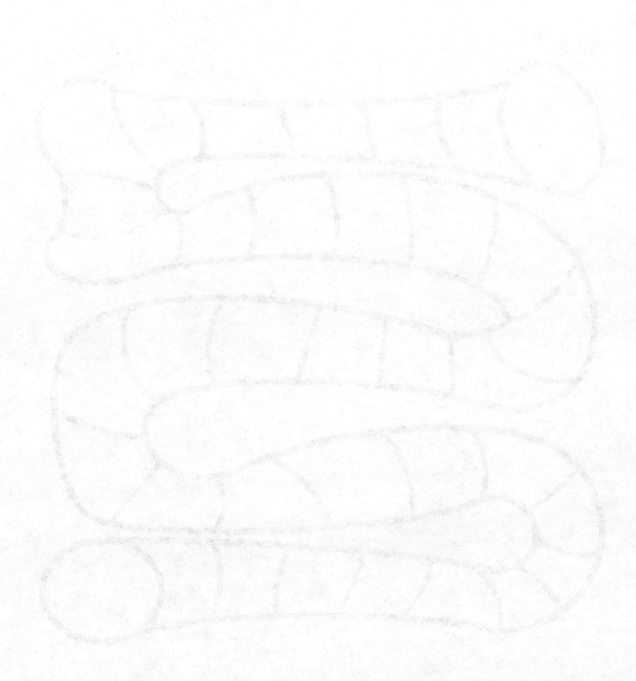

Artistic Side View

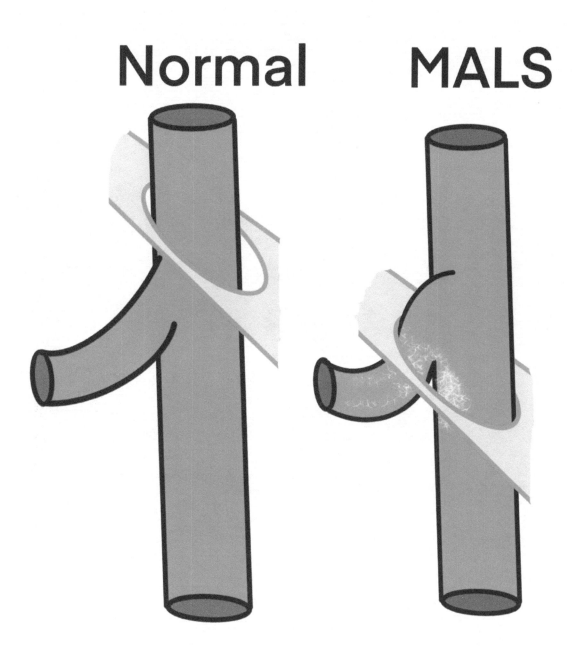

Ultrasound results will list the velocity of blood flow through the celiac artery. Higher numbers indicate that something is compressing the artery. With MALS the exhale velocity is higher. Do you have your numbers from an ultrasound?

Inhale: Exhale:

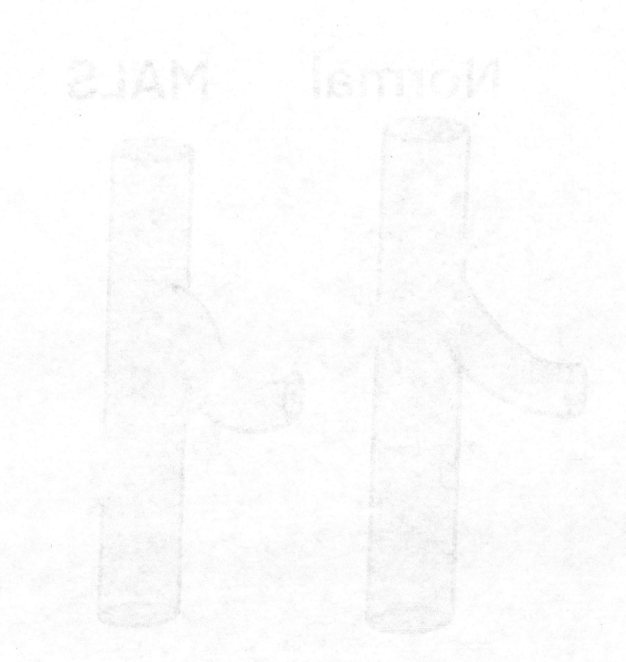

Artistic representation of MALS anatomy

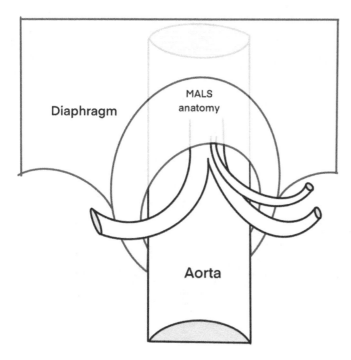

Normal anatomy

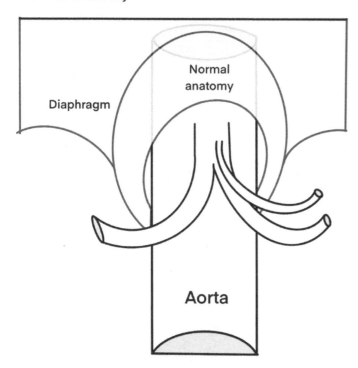

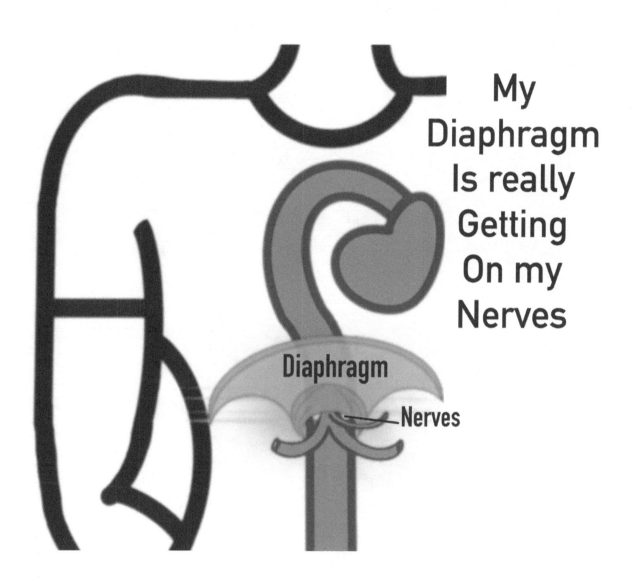

About the Author

Laurie Krause is a pharmacist who learned to flush PICC lines and start IVs before she left for work each day. She knew more about feeding tubes than the average pharmacist due to her home healthcare training to become a caregiver for her starving daughter, Makanda. Each day, she searched for the cause of her daughter's violent vomiting and stomach pain. They endured three years of vomiting, with over one hundred pounds of weight loss.

They became frustrated, emotional narrators of Makanda's story, sometimes begging for help, and some doctors were quick to judge. That's when Laurie developed the organizational forms in this workbook to share precise information promptly.

When Makanda was diagnosed in 2016, there was very little information available about MALS, so Laurie pulled out her anatomy books and made very simple drawings of the basic idea of MALS so that she could understand it better and explain it to her family. She shared her drawings on social media to help other patients and caregivers understand. She hopes that the drawing will help you with simple communication. For more precise drawings, please consult an official reference book.

Laurie lives in Seattle with her husband and a wire-haired Vizsla dog named Shaggy. Makanda and her partner live in an apartment nearby, and Makanda has a woodworking studio with a beautiful garden. You can find more information about her life after MALS at MakandaWoodshop.com.

Their complete story is in the editing phase, and they hope to publish their non-fiction story in paperback. Their struggle to find a mystery diagnosis taught them to appreciate the simple moments. But, there comes a time when you must decide to trust the doctors or question the doctors, knowing you may lose your medical team.

Each new medical team needs to be brought up to speed, so Laurie created the Maybe it's MALS Workbook.

She believes everyone knows someone with a stomach ache.

LaurieKrause.net

Made in United States
Cleveland, OH
27 June 2025